Medical Vibes from the Inside...

...things you need to Know!

PATRICIA RAYA, RN, C, MBA

CORINE A MOGENIS

ISBN 978-1-873413-39-5

MERIT PUBLISHING INTERNATIONAL

North American address:
1095 Jupiter Park Drive, Suite 7
Jupiter, FL 33458
USA

Tel: (1) 561 697 1447

Email: meritpi@aol.com

European address:
50 Highpoint, Heath Road
Weybridge, Surrey KT13 8TP
England

Tel: (44) (0) 1932 844526

Email: merituk@aol.com

www.meritpublishing.com

merit
PUBLISHING
INTERNATIONAL

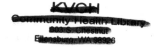

merit
PUBLISHING
INTERNATIONAL

Disclaimer: All information is for educational purposes only. The information contained in this book has been collected from highly reputable sources and presented with all due care, but we cannot warrant or represent that the information is free from all errors or omission. For specific medical advice, diagnoses, and treatment, consult your healthcare provider.

ABOUT THE AUTHORS

Patricia Raya, RN, C, MBA

Patricia (Patti) Raya, RN, C, MBA is President of PAR Enterprises: Legal Nurse Consultants www.par-nurseconsultants.com in Princeton, New Jersey. Patricia has worked in the areas of Neuroscience, High-Risk Ante-Partum Care and Risk Management. She graduated from Rutgers, The State University (New Jersey) with a Bachelor of Science degree in Management. Patricia received her Nursing degree from Raritan Valley Community College, New Jersey. She received her M.B.A. from the University of Phoenix in Arizona. Patricia has authored numerous articles published in nursing journals, and is a contributing author in Legal Nurse Consulting: Principles and Practice, 2nd Edition. She has lectured on Risk Management, Stroke Awareness, Diabetes, and Legal Nurse Consulting.

Corine A. Mogenis

Corine (Corie) Mogenis is a medical malpractice paralegal currently working for a major law firm in North Brunswick, New Jersey. Corine has almost 20 years experience working with plaintiff attorneys in case review and development. Her in-depth medical investigations have awarded her utmost respect in the legal community. Corine attended Kean University, Union, New Jersey majoring in medical laboratory technology and minoring in psychology. She received her paralegal certification from ICS, paralegal school (a subsidiary of national education corp.), Scranton, Pennsylvania. She has taken numerous continuing education classes with respect to both legal and medical issues. Corine also volunteers her time to hospice programs throughout New Jersey, as well as for the American Cancer Society and for local community charities that assist underprivileged and troubled families in those communities.

Photos by Debbie Meade and Kimberly Lewis

DEDICATIONS

Corine A. Mogenis

In Memory of my Grandmother, Natalie Chodack, whose life's difficulties, as well as her constant support, inspired me to do all I have done thus far.

To my Parents, Ray and Nancy Mogenis, for giving me the best opportunities possible in life, and to my sister, Beth Retcho and brother, Ray Mogenis, for their years of love and friendship.

To my true friend, Debbie Meade, through her friendship, love and heroic example of facing life's most difficult challenges with dignity and grace, I have been truly inspired.

To Patti Raya, not only did I get to work with the best on this project, but her humor and friendship made it all worthwhile!

And to my nieces, Nicole, Ashley and Olivia, ALL of my dear friends, colleagues, clients and hospice patients whose lives have touched mine in some deep and permanent way, I thank you all for the imprints that were left on my heart and the impact it had, which has allowed me to become the person I am today.

Patricia Raya

To my husband Alfie, whom I love dearly and truly; and who has been a steady source of encouragement, support, and back rubs. To my daughters Sharon and Kimberly, I know that you can do anything you desire. Believe in yourselves. Follow your hearts and capture your dreams. Live your lives to the fullest. You make me the proudest! I love you both 'ginormously.' Enjoy the rollercoaster of life.

For my sister Mary and brother Andrew, my niece Valerie and nephews Thomas, Brett and Kyle, I love you all, be healthy.

To Corie, I can't think of anyone I would have rather taken on this project with than you. You are a wonderful friend, and an inspiration. Thank you for helping turn this dream into a reality.

To my wonderful friend Sharon who is a mentor and a constant source of strength and motivation, thank you for everything! To my dear friend Pam, 'Don't dream it...be it.' Thank you, Rita, for your inspiration, confidence and for helping to edit this book. A special thank you to Amy, for all of your listening and reminding me to breathe. Thanks Marilyn for sharing FACTS. And finally, I'd like to thank Muriel Roberts, RN, for teaching me the art of nursing. It is from her guidance and direction that I learned not only the skills to care for my patients, but also the compassion needed to heal their souls.

Cartoon illustrations drawn by Nancy A. Mogenis. Thank you!

CONTENTS

INTRODUCTION

You are sitting in your doctor's office. The doctor has called you in because he has something to discuss. Your test results have come back and there is a problem. The hours prior to this dreaded conversation are filled with fear, anxiety and confusion. The doctor informs you that you have cancer or some other terrible illness...now what?

As the doctor continues to explain your test results, your options and the details – you sit in a daze. You can barely hear or comprehend what is being said because you are still trying to accept the very first words the doctor uttered. Thousands of thoughts run through your head as you try to figure out how to tell your family and friends, what type of doctor do you go to next, what are your specific options, the likelihood of success, how sick will you be and will this disease be the cause of your death?

This is a more common scenario than most people think. We all know someone who has been in this situation. In hindsight we all wished we had approached things differently – learned more about our illness, had researched options, doctors, and asked more questions. This book is to help prepare and inform you on how to better respond to these situations and others and to urge people to take charge of their medical care and become a vital part of their medical provider team.

At any given point in time someone, somewhere, is at a physician's office being told that they have an illness or disease. Some illnesses are relatively minor, while others will have a profound and devastating effect on the person's life. The physician will tell them about the disease, and the plan of treatment. But is this enough?

Education is the key to getting the best and most appropriate healthcare possible. This book will show you in a simple way how to become a better advocate for your own healthcare and how to take control of your medical decisions. Armed with this knowledge, you will be better prepared to understand your diagnosis, treatment options, and prognosis. This book will explain to you why information about the quality of health care is important, how to gather information about physicians and other medical providers, and how to analyze and prioritize your own health care situation. There are also sections specific to the needs of children, women's health, elder care and chapters dealing with healthcare on an international level. We have included chapters on international travel and added some sources of reference and support for the International Community as well. This book can be used as a reference tool for you, your family and your friends. Keep it handy.

CHAPTER 1

A PATIENT'S BILL OF RIGHTS, ADVANCED DIRECTIVES AND DNR

Being hospitalized is often a traumatic experience. One of the largest complaints people have is the loss of control over their environment and circumstances. As a patient, you are told when to eat, what to eat, when you are going for treatment, when your medication will be given, and even when you will be discharged home. Physicians, residents, nurses, technicians, and even students, come to you at all hours of the day and night. Ready or not, your dressing will be changed. Now, not later, they need to take some blood. Later, not now, you will get your meal. Over all, it can leave you frustrated and feeling that you lost your individuality.

Successful and efficient communication is the result of cooperation between you, the physician, the nurse, and the rest of the healthcare team. The hospital and the health care providers need to work hard in building the foundation for understanding and respect for the patient. They need to incorporate the different cultural, religious, ethnic, gender, age, disabilities and other differences in their care.

To set a precedent, the American Hospital Association developed 'A Patient's Bill of Rights.' Hospitals are encouraged to utilize this guide in providing more efficient and effective patient care. Hospitals have a copy of 'A Patient's Bill of Rights' posted in many places for patients and their families to review and understand. A copy should be posted for example, in each patient's room in a highly visible and accessible location.

PATIENT'S BILL OF RIGHTS:

In order for you to get the best practicable care, there has to be a joint effort between you and the doctors, nurses, and other members of the heath care team. Effective communication is vital in order for you to get the finest care possible. The Patient's Bill of Rights helps to contribute to more successful patient care. It does vary from state to state and is revised as needed, so it is important for you to know and understand your state's specific provisions. The language of the Patient's Bill of Rights should be easy enough for patients and their families to understand.

These Rights are summarized as follows:

- The right to receive care and services that the hospital is required by law to provide.

- The right to receive an explanation from your doctor about your condition, treatment, expected results, any risks involved in the treatment, as well as any acceptable medical alternatives.

- The right to give written consent before starting certain non-emergent medical treatments and/or procedures. Your doctor should explain to you the procedure, the risks, the recovery time, and any alternative procedures that are available. If you are not able to give informed written consent, the physician and healthcare providers will seek to obtain consent from your next of kin or guardian, or through your advanced directive (to the extent authorized by law). If the doctor is unable to obtain the written consent, he/she must document this in the medical record.

- The right to make informed decisions regarding your care. This includes the right to formulate an advance directive and to have your physician and hospital staff that provide care to you in the hospital comply with the directive.

- The right to receive information about pain, to be included in setting goals to relieve your pain and you have the right to expect a quick response if you report pain.

- The right to refuse treatment and medication (to the extent permitted by law) and to be informed of the consequences of this act.

- The right to participate in experimental research only if you give informed, written consent. You also have the right to refuse to participate in experimental research.

- The right to know the names and duties of all health care professionals providing you with care. You also have the right to know the names and functions of any outside health care agencies involved in your care and you also can refuse their participation in your care.   If needed, a translator, interpreter, or assisted listening device should be provided as soon possible.

- The right (if requested) to receive the hospital's policy and procedures regarding life-saving means, as well as the withdrawal of life support devices.   You have the right to receive in writing the rules of the hospital regarding the conduct of patients and visitors.

- The right to receive the name and phone number of the person you can ask questions about your rights or the name of the person you can complain to if you feel your rights have been violated.

- The right to access your medical record and to obtain a copy of your medical record at a reasonable fee, within 30 days after the hospital receives your written request.

- The right to receive a copy of the hospital payment rates and an itemized bill must be provided to you if requested. The hospital must answer any questions you have regarding your bill and you have the right to know if any part or your entire bill will not be covered by insurance. Also the hospital is required to help you obtain public assistance, and whatever private health insurance benefits that you are entitled to receive.

- The right to receive information from your physician and other health care providers if you need to arrange for continued health care after you are discharged from the hospital. You also have the right to have enough time before you are discharged to make the arrangements for these continued health care needs. You have the right to be informed by the hospital about the plan for appeal you are entitled to by law if you do not agree with the hospital's discharge plans.

- The right to request to be transferred to another facility, or if the transferring facility is unable to provide you with the care that you need and your physician need to provide you with an explanation for your transfer and possible alternatives.

- The right to be treated with dignity, courtesy and respect. This encompasses a storage space in your hospital room for personal use, a process in place to safeguard your personal belongings if you are unable to assume responsibility for these items and you have the right to a safe environment.

- The right to be free from physical and mental abuse, and to be free of restraints (unless they are authorized by a physician for a short period of time in order to protect your safety as well as the safety of others).

- The right for privacy during medical procedures as well as personal hygiene functions.

- The right to confidential treatment regarding your personal information.

- The right to medical treatment regardless of your age, race, religion, sex, national origin, sexual preferences, handicap, diagnosis, ability to pay or your source of payment. You have the right to exercise your constitutional rights, and your civil and legal rights.

These rights are the mechanism used to preserve the patient's values and dignity and they should be posted in patient rooms, in patient care areas, and in public places throughout the hospital. Again, please note that these rights may vary from state to state and are revised and updated as needed.

These Rights cover the hospital's responsibility to the patient. They are provided to you for your benefit and protection, so that you can have an optimal hospital stay. But what is your responsibility to the hospital? You are responsible for providing the required information necessary on insurance forms, and for paying your hospital bills, or for making arrangements for payment to the hospital. You also are responsible for cooperating with the needs of the hospital, other patients, health care workers, and other hospital employees. *Remember...effective communication between you, your family and the hospital and their staff will make your hospitalization a more positive, and more informed experience.*

ADVANCE DIRECTIVES:

An Advance Directive is a document that describes what treatment options and types of care you would like to have (or not like to have) in the event you are unable to make medical decisions. It is a legal document that becomes active when a person is unable to make or communicate their decisions. The Advance Directive will state what treatments you would or would not want. Another example of an Advance Directive is the Durable Power of Attorney (DPA). This states the person you have chosen to act as a decision maker in your health care decisions. The DPA goes into effect when you are unconscious, or are incapable of making medical decisions. *The law governing advance directives differ from state to state so it is best to be aware of the laws of your state.* If you are admitted to the hospital, a hospital representative will ask you if you have an Advance Directive. If you do not have an Advance Directive, a hospital representative can assist you with documenting your wishes as an advance directive. Your attorney can also write Advance Directives.

DNR: DO NOT RESUSCITATE:

A DNR document states that you do not want CPR (cardiopulmonary resuscitation) in the event that you stop breathing or your heart stops. A DNR will be placed on your hospital chart. DNR status is accepted in all US states.

It is important to know that you can change your mind about your Advance Directives at any time, providing you are of sound mind. If you do make changes, check your state law regarding signing and notarizing your changes. Be sure to tell your family and your doctor of any changes you decide to make.

CHAPTER 2

THE CHANGING HEALTHCARE INDUSTRY

In America, we think we have the best doctors and nurses, cutting edge technology, and highly skilled researchers. Thousands and thousands of people seek medical expertise every day. The concern most people have is how to get the best quality healthcare on a consistent basis. Patients constantly complain of receiving substandard care. The shortcomings of the healthcare system ultimately endanger the life of you, the patient.

Let's compare the two types of healthcare insurance, managed care versus traditional (or indemnity) insurance. The biggest difference is the reimbursement structure. With the traditional or fee for service insurance plan, payment is made for services rendered. Most commonly, there is a yearly deductible, and when the deductible is met, the insurance company will pay 80% of the bill. For example, if there is a $1,000 annual deductible, the first $1,000 will be paid by you, the individual, and the insurance company will pay 80% of the remaining bills for that year. You are responsible for the remaining 20% of the bills for that year.

With managed care, the insurance provider contracts with the healthcare providers for an agreed upon reimbursement for services provided. Capitation is when the managed care participating healthcare provider accepts a fixed amount of money per month. With capitation, the healthcare provider knows their monthly income, so it is beneficial for cash flow and operational budgets. A problem with capitation is that the healthcare providers are not reimbursed for routine visits. Healthcare providers need to use good judgment of services in order to increase potential profits. This is where underutilization of healthcare services can be found.

Managed care directly influences how healthcare will be provided to you, their patients. They utilize networks of providers. Managed care is criticized for providing physicians with incentives to limit care or to hold back on care. This is why patients that have the traditional or fee-for-service health care plans are more satisfied with the healthcare they receive. Interestingly, healthcare providers are also more satisfied with traditional plans than with managed care plans.

Improving the quality of healthcare is a national goal. Promoting patient safety includes reducing medication errors, reducing hospital acquired infections, improving the accuracy of patient identification, and reducing patient injury from in-hospital falls. Healthcare facilities have designed and implemented policies and procedures to address these issues to provide a safe, healing environment for patients and visitors alike.

Another way the healthcare arena is changing is the vast amount of information available to patients. Armed with information, patients are gaining control of their health care. Today, patients are researching doctors and specialists, and are 'referring' themselves, eliminating the need to go through a referring doctor. Many patients today do not consider themselves under the care of one particular doctor. Patients today are better informed, they are taking control. Because of the Internet, patients are learning about diagnostic and treatment advances at the same time as the doctors. Today's trend is for a better-informed patient that wants to take part in the decision making process as it relates to their health care.

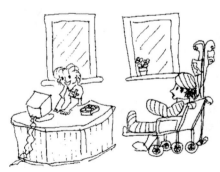

*Mr Smith - I'm <u>sorry</u> the computer says you are <u>**not**</u> a patient here - I can't help you!*

CHAPTER 3

CHOOSING ELEMENTS OF YOUR HEALTH CARE

Being able to make decisions regarding our own, or our family's health care is a great privilege and one for which we should be thankful. There are many people who do not have medical coverage and are forced to see physicians at clinics or other specified health care facilities. For those of us who are fortunate enough to have the ability to make certain decisions about our health care, we should fully utilize this choice and not take it for granted.

When purchasing your health care coverage on your own, or deciding on a choice given by an employer, making an informed decision is always advisable. Getting as much information as possible on the health care company, the physicians and hospitals that you will be able to choose, as well as details to your limitations and restrictions in the plan you select is important information to have in advance, as opposed to later on when it may be too late to do anything about it.

Begin your journey of choosing your health care coverage with the same focus, attention and detail that you would in buying a house or a car. The reason for this is that someday your life or that of a family member may depend on it!

CHOOSING YOUR MEDICAL COVERAGE

If you have the opportunity to purchase your own medical coverage or choose from a variety of companies and plans offered by an employer, you should do as much research as you can about the company. Each state has an

Insurance Commissioner. This is a state agency that governs the acts of all insurance companies that do business within that state. You can get information on these insurance companies regarding from how long they have been doing business in that state to how many complaints are pending against the company in your state.

Most insurance companies also have websites where you can find out information regarding how long they have been established, estimated costs for specific types of plans, the physicians and hospitals who participate in their plans, etc. You can also get information regarding the details of each plan. There are Health Maintenance Organizations (HMOs), Preferred Provider Organization (PPOs) and numerous categories of medical plans these days. These vary from company to company as to what your restrictions and abilities are with each plan of service. Finding out all of the details for the plan you are interested in, in advance, is key. Some plans require a referral which means you must go to your 'designated' primary care physician each and every time you have any medical problem in order to receive a referral slip that will then allow you to go to a specialist, i.e. cardiologist, dermatologist, surgeon, etc. Some plans allow you to go directly to these specialists, without a referral, but only those specialists that participate with that insurance company. A company representative can normally answer any questions you have, including those which may not be found on the website, as well as questions you have about specifics of the plan and/or physicians.

Some plans also offer prescription options. This will usually include choices of pharmacies and limitations on types of medication, costs for each medication, etc. If you take a medication, be sure to find out in advance if your local pharmacy participates in your insurance plan, and how much the insurance plan covers towards the cost of your prescription. Otherwise you can run into an inconvenient and costly outcome.

Find out what you need to know before you sign on the dotted line because that is usually the binding agreement that does not allow you to make many choices afterward.

CHOOSING YOUR DOCTOR

Choosing the doctor for you and/or your family is a crucial decision. Going

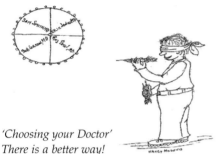

'Choosing your Doctor'
There is a better way!

to anyone in a list of medical providers given to you by the insurance company is not the way to approach this selection. If you currently have a physician that you are comfortable with, trust and have a long standing history with, you shouldn't leave that physician just because you are changing insurance companies. If you can see 'out of network' providers where it may cost you 20% or 30% of the bill as opposed to simply paying a co-payment office visit, it may be worth it.

Finding a physician you can trust and one you can rely on is not as easy as it sounds. If you opt for some random name from the book every time a new list of providers comes along, or every time you change insurance companies, this is a haphazard way of securing valuable medical care. Each time a new physician sees you, they are forced to start from scratch. If they are able to review prior medical records, they must attempt to compile a new medical profile for you and do their best to pick up where your other doctor left off. If you keep the same physician for as long as you can, it will foster a knowledgeable and secure relationship between you and your clinician. This puts you one step closer to more accurate medical care.

If you are forced to switch doctors for any number of reasons, you should attempt to investigate the doctor as best as you can before you begin treatment with him/her. Each state has a Board of Medical Examiners. This state agency governs the acts of physicians. They can tell you whether or not the doctor's license is in good standing. In some states, but not all, they can even tell you if the doctor has been sued, how many times and whether or not their license was ever revoked, if they were ever put on probation or if their privileges were limited in any way. This is all-important information to have before entrusting your life, or that of your family, to a doctor.

Don't hesitate to visit a physician's office before becoming a patient. Dropping by to see how the staff works, how polite and efficient they appear or how clean the office looks are all important in creating a comfortable environment for your medical care. Some physicians even welcome an 'interview meeting' with potential new patients. They will meet you for a few minutes to introduce themselves and explain a little about their practice and experience. This interview should help ease any fears or anxieties you have and hopefully reassure you in becoming a new patient of theirs. A physician who goes out of their way to welcome you to their practice is a caring physician and someone who is interested in your well-being.

Establishing a decent relationship with your medical providers is important. It should be approached with the same thought you give any other relationship in your life. This is an important decision.

CHAPTER 4

PREVENTING MEDICAL ERRORS

WHAT IS A MEDICAL ERROR?

A medical error is an unexpected outcome or an unexpected or wrong plan used in a patient's care. A medical error can occur in any healthcare setting, including hospitals, outpatient clinics, nursing homes, rehabilitation facilities, doctors' offices, outpatient surgery centers, pharmacies, and even at a patient's home. A medical error can include: wrong medications, surgeries, diagnosis, treatments, equipment, equipment malfunction, and erroneous lab results. Medical errors cost money, but also can cost you your life. A recent study supported by the Agency for Healthcare Research and Quality (AHRQ), found that doctors often do not do enough to help their patients make informed decisions. Uninvolved and uninformed patients are more likely to accept the doctor's choice of treatment and less likely to do what they need to do to make the treatment work [1].

HOW TO AVOID MEDICAL ERRORS

The single most important thing you can do to help prevent medical errors is to get involved in your medical care. This includes having a good line of communication between you and your doctor. The more communication, the better understanding the doctor will have for your concerns, health questions and issues, and the more your physician will explain details of your illness and treatments to you. It is important to let your healthcare provider know if you have any allergies, what medications you are taking (this includes vitamins, herbal supplements, and over-the-counter medications), medication allergies, previous surgeries, medical conditions, and family history of any medical illnesses.

When you are given a prescription for a medication, make sure the prescription is legible. Ask your doctor what the name of the medication is, and why it is being prescribed. Find out from the doctor and pharmacists what side effects are common, and get a written list of both the medication and the side effects. Make sure you know how to take the medication. That includes knowing the right time, right dose, and right route (i.e. oral, topical, injected, and rectal). Ask if there is anything that is contraindicated with the medication. For example, there are some medications that when taken, you should avoid driving, drinking alcohol, or taking other medications as they might not go well together. Some medications have food restrictions while you are taking the medication. Taking medicine incorrectly will decrease its effectiveness and it could also prove hazardous to your health.

If you are being admitted to a hospital, be sure that the hospital has experience in the area for which you need treatment. The more familiar they are with your condition, the better care you should expect to receive. Make sure that your surgeon and you agree on the part of your body to be operated on. A patient safety goal is ensuring that everyone is sure of the proper identity of the body part to be operated on. Surgeons will mark the site for identification. A 'time-out' is used in the operating room as a double check to make sure the correct area is identified.

When it is time to be discharged from the hospital, make sure that the doctor and nurse explain to you what medications have been prescribed, what physical limitations are being placed on you (for example, no driving for six weeks, no lifting of anything over 20 lbs., etc), any issues related to dressing changes or physical therapy, if a home health care provider will be needed and if so, that arrangements have been made prior to your discharge. Also, know when a follow-up visit with the doctor should be scheduled. Find out if you should be following up with additional doctors or specialists. Often, a follow-up appointment can be made at the time you are being discharged from the hospital.

Finally, take someone with you; a friend or family member who can help, ask additional questions, ask for clarification, and help ensure that everything is understood so there is minimal opportunity for medical error.

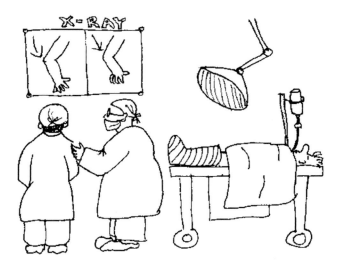

'OH.......You said ELBOW !?!

CHAPTER 5

WHAT TO DO IF YOU ARE DIAGNOSED WITH AN ILLNESS/DISEASE

Discovering that you have an illness can be one of the most devastating and confusing times of your life. There is no way to prepare for this; however your response to this news can make all the difference. Once you get past the initial shock, you can begin to get fully involved in your care by taking hold of the reins to help guide your medical decisions and treatment.

Learning as much as you possibly can by asking questions, library and Internet research will help you to understanding the information about your illness and the treatment options available. This process will allow you to play a major role in your treatment plan. This enables you to have educated discussions with your physician about your condition and all of the treatment options available to you. Together, you and your healthcare providers can decide the best choice for you.

Being told by a physician that diagnostic tests and work-ups are going to be necessary to determine what type of illness may signal your first chance to begin your search for information. There are many easy and accessible ways to search and gather information. Not only can you get information about the tests you will be having, but you can also obtain information about all of the possible illnesses that the doctor is trying to rule out. This way, when your results are in, you will have some knowledge about the illness you are diagnosed with. The knowledge you have acquired will enable you to ask appropriate questions and help you understand what to expect next.

Having a close friend or family member involved with you in your medical appointments and your decision-making is an extremely helpful plan of action. This person may understand parts of the discussions that you did not, or may ask certain questions that you didn't think to ask. By being together, you will get a better understanding of your illness and the treatments available. Trying to understand and process all of the information on your own can be overwhelming. Having another individual present will make sure that nothing is missed and that questions will be asked. Also, your friend or relative can offer emotional support, which is a huge part of making this challenging time more bearable.

Below is the first patient's case example of the above scenario:

CASE 1: Danielle E.: 'Finding a lump in your breast can be one of the scariest discoveries ever. After a routine mammography and ultrasound, I was advised to immediately seek the opinion of a breast surgeon. Since at the time of diagnosis I was very young, the thought of possible breast cancer was devastating. After discussing my concerns with Corie, one of the authors, she helped me to find medical information that indicated numerous other medical conditions, which I might have had OTHER than breast cancer. Corie accompanied me to my breast surgeon appointment where a fine-needle aspiration was performed and the doctor's opinion was rendered. Having another person there to absorb what was being said was comforting and important because as a patient, I was more involved with being frightened and anxious. She was a great support. Thankfully, a few days later, I received the call that my condition was 'benign' but would, however, require surgery. With a clear head, I was then able to go through the surgery and recover perfectly. I can't stress enough how being informed and having a support group of friends and family made all the difference in the world!'

COMMUNICATION WITH PEERS

Once you comprehend the news that you have been diagnosed with an illness, you should not be afraid to talk to others about it. You will find that you are NOT alone! Your neighbor, colleague, friend, or even an acquaintance either knows someone with the same illness, or may even have had experience with it him/or herself. This is another excellent way to obtain more information. Through discussions, you will share your concerns and feelings, and also learn more about the illness. You can find names of specialized hospitals, physicians and treatment options available. You might also learn about someone who went through what you are about to go through and came out with flying colors. Hearing these stories can give you additional support and hope, which is another key to recovery. At first, you may not want to talk about your illness with everyone. Once the initial shock wears off, you should go out and gather as much information about your illness as possible. *Remember, this is your life, so take charge of it!*

You will be surprised at how many people will be willing to help. They will help with research, finding a physician; even drive you to necessary appointments and treatments. In this time of need, people do and will reach out a helping hand to one another. It can make all the difference but if people don't know what is going on with you, they can't help.

Don't be shy. Talk about your situation, not to receive pity or sympathy but to become educated and informed. Your illness affects not only you but also many others. It is an opportunity to bring you closer to those who care about you.

GETTING INFORMATION THAT YOU NEED TO KNOW

Your initial reaction might be 'how am I going to become informed about an illness or disease? I am not a physician, nurse, or medical student. How can I get access to information, and will I be able to understand it?'

You will be surprised to hear how easy it is to access a lot of information. There is information written for the lay person and information written for those with medical understanding. All information can be obtained from hospitals, libraries, bookstores, through the Internet, and related organizations. Many of us have access to a computer with Internet capabilities either at home or at work. You can also gain Internet access from computers in libraries, colleges, and Internet cafes. Not all physicians can provide you with articles or brochures on every illness. However, once you leave the physician's office, the search for information is your responsibility. Call specific national organizations, such as the American Heart Association, the American Cancer Society, or the relevant organization to your illness. Pharmaceutical companies also have information telephone for patients, web sites or leaflets that patients can obtain for free.

How many of us do research when we are remodeling our home, buying a car, or appliance? You look into features and benefits, and make comparisons. You investigate the best brands, best prices, and the durability of products. You take time to make decisions. Then you search for the 'expert,' someone who has experience painting, remodeling, laying carpet, etc. You interview several people and check their references. You base your decision not only on the person who will give you the best price, but who you trust will be doing the best job possible.

Why don't we do this when it comes to our own health? Why wouldn't you research your illness and the treatments or surgeries you may need as carefully as you would research the types of paint and appliances you will need? We all have the power to research our condition, our illness, how much experience our physician has with treating a specific illness, how many times a physician has done a particular procedure, etc. We can choose a physician based on such information, and that in turn will add to our comfort and trust. If you put as much effort into researching your health as you would researching a new car or a contractor for home repair, you will have a wealth of knowledge and be better informed in choosing a physician to take care of you.

Getting a second opinion is ALWAYS a good idea. Especially when the diagnosis is a serious one, consulting with another physician and/or specialist is an easy way of confirming your treatment options or showing you that there may be more options available. All good physicians will welcome a second opinion.

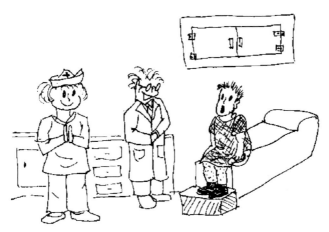

Well it's a surprise to us too 'MR' Johnson...
but the REPORT SAYS You're pregnant with TWINS!!

By seeking advice from another physician, you also broaden your treatment care providers. You can choose the physician and treatment plan that you feel is best for you and your situation. This is another opportunity for you to get involved in your care. Feeling comfortable with your doctor and the treatment options or plan of care is a key role in putting your best foot forward. It is great to know that both you and your doctor have a common goal – *getting you the best care possible with the best results!*

Insurance companies generally pay for a second opinion, as long as the physician conducting the second opinion does not share a practice with the first physician.

Patient's Case Study:

CASE 2: Darlene N.: 'After a terrible foot injury, I immediately saw a doctor. Weeks had gone by and I still had no answers or definitive treatment plan. Two different physicians had given me two differing opinions as to a diagnosis and what my follow-up care should include. One was much more drastic and aggressive than the other and I was very confused and still in a great deal of pain. When discussing this with Corie, she suggested I seek the opinion of a foot and ankle specialist. She assisted in getting me a prompt appointment and even went with me to the doctor. I was soon diagnosed with a severe foot contusion, injured ligaments and nerve damage. This clearly explained the pain and problems I was experiencing. It was further confirmed that I did NOT have any broken bones and I was spared a cast and crutches. I was completely informed about the seriousness of my injury and told that medications had to be given immediately to help reduce the swelling and aid in the healing of the injured nerves. Upon starting the medication, I soon was feeling better and was quite relieved to have received a precise medical opinion and treatment plan with a good result! I truly believe second and even third opinions are sometimes necessary. Not giving up until you get the best answer and results for yourself should always be your main objective!'

MAJOR TEACHING HOSPITALS/TREATMENT CENTERS

Hospitals and treatment centers will not only be able to provide you with some of the best treatments, but they will be able to answer a majority of your questions with certainty. A search on your illness will provide you with the names of these types of facilities, or facilities that have departments specializing in your illness.

These facilities usually host the 'best of the best' when it comes to physicians, diagnostic equipment, treatment modalities, surgical procedures and support groups. Research and medical studies are the norm. To enable doctors to improve treatment for patients, there is a constant need to learn more about various illnesses. If the standard treatments available are not considered an option for your condition, you may be a candidate for a clinical trial. The physicians, nurses, technicians, counselors, and support staff are experienced and specialized experts in treating serious illnesses and conditions, and will make your medical experience a more comfortable and reassuring one.

EXCELLENCE IN HOSPITALS:

CANCER:

University of Texas, M.D. Anderson Cancer Center, Houston, Texas
Since 1941, the Anderson Cancer Center views adult and pediatric patients by more than just their cancer symptoms. They specialize in innovative cancer treatment, cutting-edge cancer research, comprehensive education and research-based prevention of both common and rare cancers with compassion.

Memorial Sloan Kettering Cancer Center, NY
Since 1884, Sloan Kettering has been dedicated to improving the understanding and treatment of all types of cancer, both adult and

pediatric. Their dedicated team of professionals is committed solely to providing the best cancer care possible.

Johns Hopkins Hospital and Health System, Baltimore, MD
Patients at Hopkins become part of a long tradition of distinguished health care. Since their doors opened over a century ago, their mission has been excellence. Physicians there strive to lead the world in the diagnosis and treatment of disease and to train tomorrow's great physicians, nurses, and scientists. Their main focus is to always provide the highest quality health care and service to all patients.

Dana-Farber Cancer Institute, Boston, MA
Since 1947, Dana-Farber has helped adult and pediatric cancer patients by providing expert and compassionate care. Their goal is to help the patient better understand their disease, treatment, cure, prevention of cancer and related diseases.

Mayo Clinic, Rochester, MN
The Mayo Clinic is based on the idea of 'cooperative medicine.' There are teams of experts who will combine their skills and experience to help solve patient's medical problems of any type. They operate clinics and hospitals in three states and are focused on solving the medical problem – whatever it may take.

CARDIOLOGY:

Cleveland Clinic, OH
The Cleveland Clinic has a long outstanding history in treating a multitude of cardiac diseases from the simple to the extremely complex.